SCRATCHING BENEATH THE SURFACE...

SCRATCHING BENEATH THE SURFACE…

What can hypnotherapy do for you?

Jeff Hutchens

To order additional copies of this book, contact:
www.lulu.com

CONTENTS:

Introduction: From the voice of a hypnotherapist

As a hypnotherapist I have come to understand the subconscious, as it is where the work takes place and the focus of each session. A key factor in the need for hypnosis as part of the therapy is because of the CCF – the conscious critical faculty – which is the filter between our conscious mind and our subconscious. The subconscious takes on messages from a young age that are largely stored as facts and become the basis of our belief system – the 'rules' that we give ourselves to live by. If these messages have been positive and affirming then there is a strong chance that we will live in the benefit of this positive subconscious basis for our lives – we will 'believe' in ourselves, as they say. If the opposite has happened, then we will tend to believe only the negative about ourselves. In this way our CCF will seek to compare what we hear on a day to day basis with our internal belief system – it will accept or reject things based on this. For example, I have been told from a young age that I cannot do maths, that I come from a long line of people in our family that can't do maths, and that I will never amount to anything in school, and should avoid any careers to do with maths, accounting, possibly even money. This message will have come from a number of sources, and perhaps include experiences that reinforce my inner belief. Perhaps some kind teacher then chooses to tell me that I could be good at maths and that I should try harder in school. At this point my CCF will filter this new message from my teacher in the light of what I already believe about myself – and will naturally reject it out of hand – it could not possibly be true; the teacher must not have understood how bad I am at maths!

'We're terrible at realising what goes on in other people's heads because we are trapped inside our own'
Derren Brown

Are you trapped in your own world of negativity? Are you struggling to work out how other people seem to manage when you find things so hard? Are you wanting to find a powerful release into confidence and success? Are you weighed down with anxious thoughts that stress you out and make you angry?

It happens to so many of us – we get trapped inside our own heads and can't see a way out of the negative cycles that our thought patterns have created for us. It may be a specific traumatic event that has long been forgotten by your conscious mind that could be holding you back. It may be a series of events that seemed smaller and unconnected in your conscious mind – each one seemingly insignificant – but remembered as a pattern by your subconscious mind and causing a reaction that shows itself in any similar feeling in the present that becomes anxiety, panic, loss of confidence, or even anger and fear. It seems that everyone else has 'got it together' when you try your over-practiced 'mind-reading' skills, and you crush your hopes by presuming that you are the only one who is at a loss; when in reality, many are in the same position as you and trying to figure it out in their own silence. But for you now, you are ready for transformation…you are ready to make some changes in your subconscious mind through the power of hypnotherapy and NLP and find the release that you have always wanted. When you receive a course of hypnotherapy you will find the release that you really want and will find a way of understanding what is going on in your head – and maybe even a little more about others too; as long as you promise to give up your mind-reading habit! It is time for your transformation and it will make all the difference when you start…so what is stopping you?

My job as a hypnotherapist is to relax a client, to gain access to the subconscious whilst they are in a trance state, so that they can by-pass their CCF and allow some positive suggestions and affirmations to be placed into their subconscious to counteract the negative beliefs and realign them with the positive possibility that they can be good at maths, in this instant, and that they don't have to live in the negativity of the prior messages and beliefs. The subconscious works to accept the new suggestions as the CCF is now out of action, and in this state of trance a client is to find a new set of beliefs that will allow them to live with a new positive mind-set that will allow them to achieve in whatever area of life they are having problems in prior to the therapy.

Hypnosis can be seen as a natural state of mind also known as a trance which is brought about by a set of hypnosis techniques, largely based around relaxation, a state which opens up a person to suggestions through access into the subconscious mind which comes to the fore during a state of relaxed trance. In a state of hypnosis, you are able to take on board these suggestions for positive change in your life and notice real positive transformation in the areas of your life where you need it most. Now, don't get me wrong, it is important that you are actively seeking these positive changes, and open to the suggestions and the idea of hypnosis – therefore you cannot be hypnotised against your will, and cannot do anything that will contravene your true selves and values, and it is therefore very safe for you to undergo.

> 'Allow yourself to see what you don't allow yourself to see' **Milton Erickson**
>
> Are you ready for some self-revelation? Are you willing to dig deep and release the negativity of the past emotional blocks that are holding you back? Are you wanting to discover your inner strengths and unleash their power?
>
> The subconscious mind holds depths of insight and knowledge that controls how you are handling life. Events and experiences are stored away from before your birth, and your subconscious remembers

everything. I have worked with people who have unlocked memories of emotional trauma at birth or just after. Others who can recall with absolute clarity experiences from childhood that had long been repressed to 'keep them safe'; unfortunately, these can become the *sanskaras* that hold a person back in the present and affect their confidence, stress and anxiety levels, and even create fears and phobias. Healing is available when these experiences are unlocked as an adult, allowing freedom from the past. When you let yourself 'see' these things then release and wholeness is possible.

So, what can hypnotherapy do for you?

- You can see what has been hidden from you, and locked inside where your younger 'you' hides away worried, anxious or in fear

- You can bring healing to your inner child and unlock their traumatic experiences, their emotional hurts, and find new strength from the inside out

- You can take on board positive thoughts to replace the negativity

- You can allow yourself the privilege of reinventing yourself and starting over – freeing yourself to live the life you always wanted

The state of hypnosis is a natural state for all humans, where a person enters a trance of some kind and they work on autopilot as the subconscious is in charge. It could happen in many areas of a persons' life, for example, when driving a car a person will arrive at a destination and not be consciously aware of the journey, as they were daydreaming while their subconscious took over in an automatic way, so that they were able to drift off into a state of trance as their thoughts were anywhere other than concentrating on driving. For me, I have this kind of thing whilst out jogging, when my conscious mind will drift off into problem solving mode, or sometimes creative mode, as my subconscious is in charge of the muscle action and rhythm of my running, and I run on autopilot for a time – until I need to cross a road, when my conscious mind alerts me to potential hazards, and I am back in the 'real world' once again. It is believed that you spend about 80% of your day in trance states – it is *that* natural!

Part one: How does hypnotherapy work and what can it help with?

How does hypnosis work?

When the subconscious is in charge and you are in a state of hypnosis or trance, then it seems that you are more open to suggestions which can alter your mind and bring change from deep within and allow for the possibility of behaviour modification. In this state of hypnosis under the guidance of a hypnotherapist, you can easily find ways to unblock psychological problems on a subconscious level to affect real change in your everyday life, bypassing the conscious thoughts that may not understand the source of the problem. From a science point of view, it is possible to measure the changes in brain waves. The four measurable waves go from the alert state of 'beta', through the more relaxed state of 'alpha' which is more creative, on into the deep trance state of 'theta', and finally into 'delta' which is a deep sleep. You are more suggestible, and open to change in the states of alpha and theta, as well as the deep sleep of delta. However, for the hypnotherapist the most 'useful' states are perceived to be alpha and theta, although it must be recognised that individuals respond to suggestion in different ways and some might be more suggestible in a moderate trance state whilst others will have little suggestibility even in the deeper states – it really depends on you. In this state of hypnosis you may experience relaxation or sleepiness – this is a fabulous part of the therapy; it is all about the relaxation!

Even though a person can be in a trance state when not relaxed, such as the focused athlete on the starting blocks who is able to remove the outside influences in their absolute concentration to achieve their goals, relaxation is an important element of the trance required for hypnotherapy. This is because during hypnosis the person is obtaining a state that exhibits selective attention, increased suggestibility and a special state of consciousness which is achieved through deep relaxation.

Trained in relaxation techniques a hypnotherapist can encourage you to enjoy a beautiful time of relaxation and healing through the process of hypnotherapy – and all of my clients enjoy this as part of the process; it is healing in and of itself.

> 'The unconscious mind records all 1001 little details the conscious mind neglects' **John Grinder**
>
> The unconscious mind knows everything about you. It remembers everything that you have ever done, and everything that you have experienced since before birth. It holds all of your secrets. It holds all of your repressed memories that it has attempted to keep safe to protect you from harm at the time…but they are still there – leaking hurt and harm like toxic waste buried in the earth. The poisonous gases find a way of seeping to the surface bringing with them the often-deadly substances causing harm to those who are live in affected areas. The toxicity doesn't go away just because it is out of sight – or in the

case of repressed memories; out of mind. The only way to deal with buried toxic waste is to dig it up and release it before finding ways of safely disposing of it.

A great and powerful way to release repressed memories that are full of toxic emotional trauma and negative experiences, is through 'digging them up' safely through hypnotherapy. Each one of those '1001' experiences could hold you back, causing anxiety, fear, worry and poisoning your confidence from deep inside. They might lead to a phobia; they might be the cause of weight problems or other addictions. We are complex beings and our past can hold the clues to our future if we are prepared to play detective through the power of hypnotherapy. Re-visiting our younger impressionable selves to heal the memories and undermine their power and influence over us can be the key to unlock our issues.

What can hypnotherapy help with?

- **Anxiety and panic attacks**

Hypnotherapy works in a number of ways with anxiety. Firstly, by removing and particular source of the anxiety. Often your subconscious stores negative emotional reactions from your past and links this to present situations or anticipation of the future. When these memories are unlocked, faced, dealt with and then released – then the anxiety in the present and future loses its power and becomes manageable once again. It may be that negative thought patterns have grown up over the years, rather than resulting from a single event, and hypnotherapy can help with the re-programming of the mind into a positive state that can cope with and then thrive in new situations.

- **Confidence**

A lack of confidence may be the result of a lack of self-belief after years of self-doubt and a questioning of your ability and this can be addressed by building in confident thought patterns through hypnotherapy and allowing the negative patterns to be replaced through the process of hypnotherapy. This may also be the result of a single trauma which can be released through dealing with this past event and its memory imprint on the subconscious. When linked with NLP coaching and some CBT, you can find new situations to build your confidence for the future as you set bigger goals and achieve them to prove the new thought processes in the future. This is building success on success for a powerful transformation.

- **Anger**

Anger issues are often rooted in the past. As well as anger release coaching to clear the channels, it may be a trauma that is causing the hang-ups in a particular area from a memory in the subconscious mind. When revisited through hypnosis, this can be released, dealt with and healed to allow a more controlled anger response that is important for achievement of change in your life. This is good anger that provides a motivation in a positive way and allows for your assertive self to deal with situations and build your confidence in times of conflict. Negative anger must be released first to allow positive anger to be of any use for you.

• Fears and phobias

By definition, irrational fears and phobias are of the mind; the subconscious mind where the programme running your reactions has become damaged by some kind of trauma – usually from early childhood – and stored so that it triggers an over-reaction to particular situations. The original trauma may have nothing to do with the actual phobia but is connected by the subconscious in a way that makes sense to it as it tries to 'protect' you from harm. Of course, there is no real danger – if it were that would not be a phobia; just common sense! I have no intention of curing your phobia of poisonous snakes when you should be running! Releasing the trigger and then reinforcing the subconscious mind with confidence messages serves to change the phobic response and irrational fear. Sometimes NLP can help here with powerful reprogramming occurring under a state of hypnosis to transform the negative feelings attached to a particular memory in the conscious mind that is being triggered by the subconscious memory. Hypnotherapy can help support you in dealing with the fears and phobias though it must be noted that each person is different, and you will take on the re-programming when you are ready to release your phobia from your life and let go of any other gains you might be making through the fear.

- **Weight loss**

Hypnotherapy is fabulous for weight loss in a number of ways. Some people like the hypno gastric band which is a non-invasive surgery to restrict their eating altogether. For others, reprogramming can help them cut the cravings and learn new positive eating patterns, finding ways to look for healthy options and smaller portions as the positive messages are taken on board in the subconscious and new body images are visualised to empower the process of weight loss. Sometimes there may be a trigger anchored in their past that has created negative associations with food that can be released and dealt with as the memory is revisited. Maybe a person is struggling with exercise and the psychology of getting going, and the NLP coaching and reprogramming can create a positive mindset, which brings powerful support to the hypnotherapy process to allow complete transformation.

- **Quitting smoking**

Hypnotherapy is a powerful treatment for the addiction to cigarettes by allowing you to visualise being smoke-free, engaging your imagination to stimulate the desire for change, and initiating new programming for the mind to overcome the cravings to allow a healthy and positive transformation in your life. This is recommended on the list of resources by the NHS.

> 'Hypnosis is the most effective way of giving up smoking, according to the largest scientific comparison of ways of breaking the habit' **New Scientist**
>
> 'I should have done it years ago. It's amazing I didn't want cigarettes anymore' **Matt Damon** on hypnosis

- **Fibromyalgia and other conditions**

Whilst hypnotherapy would not claim to have the ability to heal a person of a condition, it is fabulous for dealing with the many symptoms. Hypnotherapy can support pain management, help with sleep deprivation, provide stress relief, and bring relaxation. These symptoms can be in place in other conditions, and so hypnotherapy is not limited to fibromyalgia, and indeed as mentioned, has been used over the years as an anaesthetic by turning off the pain receptors through the power of the subconscious mind.

'People don't' come to therapy to change their past, but their future' **Milton Erickson**

You want a better future? Who doesn't? Focusing on that better future will inspire you, allow you to dream and set lofty goals, and encourage you to begin to take action towards your amazing fulfilled life. Coaching is a fabulous way to get the best out of your journey to your stress-less life.

So why are you contemplating therapy? Why is hypnotherapy part of your journey to success? What can hypnotherapy do for you?

The past can hold you back from your future. Fact. When you have experienced difficult events, maybe even traumatic events, they leave an emotional impression on

---

your subconscious. A dark stain if you will. Any other experiences that feel similar will add weight to the buried memory, and the over-reactions of an underdeveloped set of childhood emotions leave an impression of negativity become a habitual learned behaviour that outworks itself in anxiety, worry and a sense of questioning and lack of self-belief and assurance. For many, they stumble on through, ignoring the inner voice, they set goals and wonder why they fail to make any progress. They are debilitated and hampered from somewhere deep inside and are baffled and self-berating to the point of frustration. All of this reinforces that self-doubt as negative thoughts build on previous negativity to create a recipe for continuous failure. It feels like a perpetual battle that they can never win. They become depressed and hopeless; worry turned in on itself, and they feel incapable on every level. For a few others they realise that there is a power in hypnotherapy and seek release from their past so that they can go full steam ahead with their future journey of success: they learn to free themselves to live a stress-less life.

It is time for a dramatic release from your own past that is holding you back. It is time for transformation from the inside out. Hypnotherapy and coaching are a powerful combination; a formula for your best possible success. It is time to find yours.

The hypnotherapy process – what can I expect?

In essence: Lots and lots of relaxation! Each session will allow you to find the time to gain a deep state of relaxation that allows your conscious mind to switch off from being in charge and allow your subconscious to get to the forefront. You are then more receptive to positive suggestions that can bring about the transformation that you desire. It won't go against your moral principles and if any conflict occurred you would either reject the suggestion, or, more likely, awaken and question the hypnotherapist much like you are snapped back from trance when driving if the tail-lights of the car in front come on as a warning. You know that feeling – if you are a driver it probably happens every time you drive. Thus, hypnotherapy works *with* your goals and desires, and so a part of session one would involve setting your goals for the course of hypnotherapy. This would be followed by relaxation and trance inducement, followed by a 'script' of positive messages into your subconscious mind. You may be aware of the whole session; never go deeper than alpha brainwaves to give you the science! Or you may feel like you drift in and out of awareness of the hypnotherapists voice. At the end of the script you will be awakened and feel refreshed and rested as if from a long sleep.

In session two there may be the opportunity to establish any past causes or triggers and some investigation may take place looking for clues in the subconscious, and this would be followed by another script to reinforce the positive messages once again.

In session three you may revisit relevant memories and find deep healing in a number of ways as you allow for transformation from your triggers in the past, followed by messages of confidence and positivity.

The following sessions would reinforce the confidence with relaxation and scripts of positivity and confidence to allow you to fill up any negative spaces left with positive reinforcement to secure a confident successful future.

Another session is recommended around a month later to reinforce the whole process and bring it to a conclusion. If any coaching is required to help shape the future based on the new-found confidence a person has, then this will be set up from this session onwards to provide support into the future. It may be that NLP reprogramming may form part of any of the hypnotherapy sessions, and the creation of the positive mindset through coaching also builds in the principles of NLP for powerful transformation.

'The easier you can make it inside your head, the easier it will make things outside your head' **Richard Bandler**

The garden was a mess. There was an accumulation of broken toys, tools, garden waste and a ridiculous overgrowth of weeds and shrubs. The garden seemed small, claustrophobic, dirty and generally a place to avoid rather than to spend time enjoying the outburst of early summer sun.

After a week of hard work by a variety of contributors including some professionals, the garden seemed twice its size. It felt airy and expansive – fresh, healthy and inviting. Sitting enjoying a cold beer on a summer evening seemed entirely possible again. It was a transformation.

Negative thoughts and emotional blocks can feel a bit like the overgrown and cluttered garden in our minds sometimes. There is no room for anything positive, as all thoughts are choked by the negativity any time they start to grow. Add to that the rubbish dumped on top by others who love to give their 'realistic' advice, and it can feel like a mess of unclear thinking that leaves us feeling trapped and claustrophobic. The inside of our head is cluttered and stifling, leaving us feel weighed down, anxious, depressed, lacking confidence or even making us angry with ourselves and the life we feel we are stuck with.

It is possible to clear this yourself; but it takes a lot of time and effort and it can leave you tired and wasted, and some is impossible to shift at all. When you allow yourself to hire in a professional, as I had to do to get a large tree removed from the garden, everything gets done quicker and so much more efficiently and effectively.

Hypnotherapy can allow you a subconscious detox and cleanse. Coaching can allow you to plan for the future and fill up your head with positive thoughts that are clear and focused.

The gardener has plans for a beautiful space that is ordered and organised into a place that is inviting and peaceful. There will be no clutter or wasted space. It will be the way the garden was always intended to be. You too can become the person you were intended to be; with no negativity holding you back; with positive, confident thought processes that allow you to unleash your potential for success in your life. The time for transformation is now.

Part two: A little history and science - where did it all come from and why?

Although hypnosis dates way back into history with experiences reported in ancient Egypt, in Australia amongst the Aborigines, as well as Native American and Hindu cultures; modern hypnotherapy can perhaps be more readily traced to the work of a few practitioners from the 18th century onwards. The 'animal magnetism' of Franz Mesmer certainly had an influence, believing that the fluids inside a person could be manipulated by magnets, Mesmer created therapy based on this theory and even reportedly cured a blind girl in 1777 but was accused of magic by the girl's father. He later ditched the magnets for iron rods protruding from a tub of hot water. Strange though it may seem, this is linked to hypnosis and the subconscious as it was later surmised that it was the belief of the person that brought about the changes and in fact they were in a kind of trance for this to take place (thus the term 'mesmerised' which we associate with this kind of experience today).

The term 'hypnosis' was first used in 1840 by physician James Braid (1795-1860), based on the Greek god of sleep 'hypnos' and the term has stuck, despite it being slightly misleading as the person being hypnotised is not actually asleep – most of the time! It is believed that around this time Dr. James Esdaile (1808-1859) was working in India and managed to perform nearly four hundred successful operations using hypnosis in place of any pharmaceutical anaesthetic. This technique was also used around the same time by Dr John Elliotson (1791-1868) for operations, and once in front of around two hundred medics as they watched him perform an operation to show off this in practice. Reminds me of the viewing room in Greys' Anatomy – but the reality may be more like the observations in the Frankenstein film with Kenneth Brannagh! Auguste Leibeault (1823-1904) provided treatments for the poverty-stricken people of France and is reported to have cured a patient of sciatica, and together with Hippolyte Bernheim (1837-1919 - created the idea of scripts that are still used in clinical hypnosis today. Sigmund Freud studied under Leibeault and Bernheim before rejecting hypnosis in favour or Free Association and dream interpretation later in his work – perhaps this allowed hypnosis to blend into the background for a time as the psychology took precedent once Freud had gained his reputation, however, his link is significant nevertheless to the history of hypnotherapy as he made important contributions to work of hypnotherapy in the early 1890's and his views on the power of the unconscious mind and its influence on his clients was discovered during his work with hypnosis. A French neurologist took up the mantle finding many healing effects of the use of hypnosis around the turn of the twentieth century. In 1932 Milton Erickson was born and would become known as the 'father of modern hypnosis' with his work on 'indirect suggestion' and his use of storytelling as part of his methods and he would go on the influence Richard Bandler and John Grinder in the creation of NLP and their developments in the late 1970's building on the work of hypnotherapy through the centuries.

> 'Thought can be so seductive and hypnotic that it absorbs your attention totally, so you become your thoughts' **Eckhart Tolle**

It seems to be true that we become what we think about. When we focus all of our thoughts on something, we become consumed by it; it takes over who we are, and we get what we wish for. It this is true, then it makes sense to be careful what we think about, be sure to focus on what we really want. As the saying goes 'be careful what you wish for'.

This can be a cycle of negativity if we fail to take control of our thought processes and turn them into a powerhouse of positive focus for our lives.

The setting of goals based on our dreams can be the first step on this journey to harness the power of becoming what we think about.

So, what is it that you want? Really want? Take time to write it down in detail and clarity, and then focus on this every day. Then do one thing each day to move towards your goal. You have to get active. Take back control of your thoughts and then your actions. Begin to live the stress-less life.

Part three: Stress-less hypnotherapy in action – a few cases in point...

Matthew

Matthew came to me regarding his lack of confidence, but it quickly became apparent that there were more issues going on. He did indeed have issues with confidence, but this had led him to feel inferior in his life and in particular in his approach to relationships. He had gone from bad partner choice to worse partner choice - always seeking after something that was never there. His low self-esteem that was linked to this poor confidence and bad judgement, meant that he would put up with the worst behaviour from his partners. He would stay in relationships that were bordering on the abusive, just so that he could be with someone rather than be alone. The worst part was he was able to recognise his patterns of poor choices in relationships – yet time and again opened himself up to abuse by preferring to be with someone who 'wasn't perfect' as he justified it to himself, as he had such a fear of being alone which terrified him.

Through hypnotherapy, Matthew was able to work on himself from the inside out. The process began with some clinical hypnotherapy to begin to reinforce some confidence in the subconscious to support the process. After a few weeks he was ready to tackle some of the bigger issues from his past, and was able to journey back to the start of it all and understand how issues of the way he was treated in childhood had a bearing on his confidence in his life and relationships, and how he could allow himself to be treated badly each and every time as a result. Through some inner child healing, Matthew was able to find release from the issues behind his self-esteem and lack of confidence, as he let them go and opened himself up to love all parts of himself as they were reunited in healing. Over the next few sessions his confidence was reinforced, and he found he had the confidence to let go of a toxic relationship and found he was contented in who he was and made some decisions to wait until he was ready for a partner who was 'worthy of him' as he put it.

He stated: 'Through hypnotherapy I received a powerful release from my past, which shocked me as I was very wary of the idea of being hypnotised and was cynical that it could have any effect for me. Once I decided to give it a go, I found the experience affected me deeply; I feel totally transformed – something which I never thought was possible. I am a new man. It is amazing how powerful hypnotherapy was for me, I would never have believed it before I gave it a try'

'You use hypnosis not as a cure but as a means of establishing a favourable climate in which to learn'
Milton Erickson

Why hypnotherapy? Why not just counselling, coaching or psychotherapy?

When it comes down to it, it's all about relaxation. This is why hypnotherapy is such a fabulous and powerful form of therapy. It is also a relaxation session. As a teacher I noticed that teenagers learn easily when they are having fun – well I was a drama teacher! And I believe that fun and relaxation go hand in hand. In a state of relaxation, our learning defences are down and we take on board information easily and readily. We are such natural learners when we are relaxed, interested and engaged – when we are having fun. Conversely, when we try to 'study hard', we clam up, sweat, force concentration and try to squeeze information into a reluctant and stressed out mind – it feels closed off and learning seems so difficult.

If we are 'trying hard to change' in therapy, we can end up closing ourselves off as a result of trying too much, and it takes a long time of sustained effort to affect any kind of transformation.

In hypnotherapy the person is relaxed, the mind is enjoying stories and is able to unwind and go with the flow of the voice of the storyteller. Defences are down, and positive messages of change and transformation are taken on readily and easily. When you relax and allow it to happen, learning is quicker and effortless – just think about that favourite song of yours that you know all the words to- without ever 'trying' or 'studying hard' to learn them. What about your favourite comedy show that you recite your favourite scenes from with your friends? All relaxed learning can be as easy and effortless as this, and hypnotherapy creates the perfect climate for learning those positive changes that you wish to make for your successful life. If you are ready for some serious change, allow hypnotherapy to create the climate for your learning journey and transformation in your life.

Hannah

'I was desperate to find a way of getting to my target weight. I had tried all of the fad diets and had been a classic "yo-yo" for years, as I jumped straight back up to beyond my original weight once the diet was over. It was really getting me down and affecting my confidence in a big way. I saw myself as unlovable and gross, and I wanted to give up on everything at one point. When I saw the advert for hypnotherapy, I was at the point where I would try anything – nothing more than that really; I had lost all hope that anything could work for me. The first thing that I noticed was that my snacking desires had gone. I mean it was amazing. I could actually walk past the chocolate in the supermarket, and it was as if it wasn't there and I had no desire to buy it let alone eat it. I didn't miss it, that was the weird thing – even the mini-eggs around Easter time. I literally had no need for it anymore. This was shocking to me, as they were "my thing"; my *vice* of choice up until this point. If I'm honest, it was the snacking that was holding me back, and I noticed that pretty soon I had managed to shift a couple of pounds each week, and this gave me the momentum to keep going. I received some coaching at this point to allow me to set up some serious goals for the next steps, and the hypnotherapy was there to reinforce to positive images of the "new me" that I started to visualise. The rest is history, and I have never looked back. I am pleased with the results and I know that this time I am going to sort out my life and confidence to suit the new me that I have become. It feels so good!'

Working with Hannah was a great experience. She was motivated to get going on her weight loss and used the hypnotherapy to work in line with her goals, and gain momentum to get started from the inside out. We looked at the idea of the hypno-gastric band and some exercise as part of the package as she set herself some goals for overall life changes as the hypnotherapy worked from the inside out. In the end she didn't take up the gastric band as she was making the progress that she wanted; along with the exercise, she changed her eating habits – no more snacking - and got a handle on the portion size and ended up going beyond her targets and making herself very proud.

'Hypnosis is to consciousness what a telephoto lens is to a camera' **David Spiegel**

When I was twelve, I bought my first SLR camera and I was about to get serious about photography. Well, the twelve-year-old version of serious! I wanted all the gear; I wanted to learn to develop my own pictures; I wanted a telephoto or zoom lens; I wanted close up filters. But I was twelve and I had used up all of my money from Christmas, birthdays and savings to buy the camera. At that age a telephoto or zoom lens was way out of my price range and it would be years before I could add one to my camera. My photography was limited by my lack of equipment. Fortunately for me it snowed that year – very heavily. Six-foot snow drifts everywhere, and metre long icicles hanging just outside my own window. I could take pictures of the obvious; of the easy access things that were apparent to everyone – and I had some great photos – but I couldn't look any further or photograph the more out of reach things. I was limited to my own visual perspective.

Without the telephoto lens of hypnotherapy, you will only notice the obvious things that your conscious mind has always been aware of. You will only have access to your usual memories and won't be able to look any further at the out of reach things that are holding you back from your subconscious. You will only 'scratch the surface' of your issues and will perhaps go with the obvious, shallow solutions.

Hypnotherapy allows you to go deep, to get to the heart of the issue and deal with the root cause. This will allow meaningful and lasting change as the power of your past hurts and traumas is removed from the source of the pain. This allows healing and deep change from the inside out. This is the transforming power of hypnotherapy. It acts like the telephoto lens and empowers you to go beyond the usual to the best solution. It allows you to release yourself from the blocks and discover your wow!

Amelia

Amelia came to me because she was struggling with anxiety. The focus was work at the time, and she was worried that she was not able to cope with all that she was being asked to do. As a teacher she felt that the job was becoming overwhelming for her, and she never felt as if she could do enough to keep up, and always was 'playing catch up' as she put it. On top of this her family circumstances were difficult as her mother was dying of cancer, slowly and painfully. Her mother was the kind who would never ask for help if she needed it; but would drop passive-aggressive hints that were laden with guilt. As Amelia was living far away from her mum she also felt that whatever she did was, once again, 'never enough'. Amelia had begun letting all of this affect her self-esteem and felt that she herself was not 'enough' and she was feeling low and 'stuck' in a horrific downward spiral of negativity which seemed impossible to get out of. It is interesting how many times anxiety and depression are linked in a person's life – I see it time and again – and for Amelia this was a combination that led her to feel powerless and overwhelmed by her life. I remember her in tears as she talked of her feelings of inadequacy and self-doubt.

Through the process of hypnotherapy, we uncovered a few of her triggers from the past which allowed her to be ready for taking on confidence from the inside out as she felt the reinforcement of her self-esteem from the inside out through the power of her subconscious. With wrap-around coaching to set her up for the future with confidence building goal achievement she was well on her way to living a life that was thriving rather than surviving as Wayne Dyer would have said. It is with clients such as Amelia who are struggling with self-confidence, anxiety, stress and overwhelm, that hypnotherapy proves so transformational for as they literally reinvent themselves from the foundation of the subconscious up into every area of their lives, and it is a privilege to be a part of their journey on the road to healing and success.

Amelia: 'Before working with Jeff I was literally a mess! I was down on myself all of the time and felt that there was no way out of this cycle of negative energy that was really getting to me. I thought that I had tried everything, and although the counselling helped a little, I still questioned who I was and couldn't find a way out. The relaxation of the hypnotherapy was a tonic in itself and a definite benefit of the process for me. Through hypnotherapy I was able to visualise a new version of myself that I could be happy with and started to see that I could a success – having thought that I would be happy just coping with my life. I am so much more than that, I am definitely enough, and I feel that through the process of hypnotherapy I lost my negative past experiences and found a version of myself that I really like. It was, as Jeff would say, *transformational*!'

'Hypnosis seems helpful in treating addictions, and the depression and anxiety associated with them'

Psychology Today

'It is hard to find a field that hasn't used hypnosis successfully, everything from quitting smoking to IBS'

Good Morning America

It is fabulous when the power of hypnotherapy is backed up by the respected associations such as the in the world of psychology and the popular media which can often be particularly scathing of the alternative medicine realm. Of course, many forget that hypnotherapy predates the practice of psychology, psychotherapy, counselling, CBT and even NLP. It was originally important as a non-pharmaceutical method of anaesthetic when it was discovered how powerful the subconscious could be in the treatment of the body and its ailments. It was found that it could help manage pain, deal with pain, and even stimulate healing from deep within the body. Hypnotherapy can stimulate the body's natural healing mechanisms and stem the flow of the negative impulses of disease, as well as bring the more obvious healing to mental health conditions that are firmly based in the mind. Anxiety, issues of self-confidence and self-image, fears and phobias, addictions to cigarettes, drugs and alcohol, as well as help the body self-regulate in terms of cravings and over-eating in the process of weight loss. More recent conditions such as fibromyalgia have found huge benefits from hypnotherapy in terms of pain management, relaxation therapy, stress relief and sleep deprivation. This has seen inroads in dealing with irritable bowels – IBS – and much more. Hypnotherapy is recognised by the NHS for it's hypnobirthing and its dealing with fibromyalgia, which shows how far things have come – particularly as they refuse to embrace counselling as a profession, seeing it as a secondary therapy rather than on the frontline. Is it time for your transformation through hypnotherapy - even from your medical condition?

Jackie

'Powerful stuff! That is the phrase that came to mind when working with Jeff in his hypnotherapy room. I have such pleasant memories of my time in that therapeutic space. I was able to release some of my anxiety through opening up some of my memories, including a particularly healing experience when I was able to resolve issues regarding my late mother. I found that I could walk a little lighter after the powerful release from my past that I experienced. I noticed how this affected my levels of confidence, and how I was so much more able to take things in my stride after my hypnotherapy. Things that had a been a big deal before the therapy I was able to handle and just get on with it in a confident way and my anxiety issues melted away. It was truly incredible and such a healing time for me which was so powerful for me that I know I have changed in ways that I had no idea were possible before the therapy. I would thoroughly recommend this for anyone; what have you got to lose but your hang-ups?!'

My time with Jackie was very precious to me. She truly engaged thoroughly with the hypnotherapy process; used the resources I gave her; and found a huge amount of healing through the process. She valued the process in ways that truly blessed me as I was encouraged by the amazing progress that she made week on week. It was early on in my career and I really needed to know how powerful that hypnotherapy could be – and Jackie proved this to me; the theories worked, and I was determined to bring this powerful transformation to as many people as would benefit from it. Without Jackie, I would not be as far along as I am today – and I am truly grateful and blessed to work with such fabulous clients. They make this all worthwhile!

'Studies show that people who combine diet and exercise with hypnosis lose more weight than they do with diet and exercise alone' **Allure**

Hypnotherapy is powerful when it comes to weight loss and weight management. It may be through the power of positive messages in the subconscious changing attitudes to food; it may be the power of the relaxation that allows the body to take on board changes so readily; it may be that they are released from their negative past emotional attachments to food as they drift back into their past memories to find true healing; it may be from the hypno gastric band – a non-invasive 'surgery' that allows the subconscious mind to lessen the amount of food a body can take in; it may be finding a mindset that is supported from the subconscious finally working for their goals; but hypnotherapy works powerfully for weight loss. It is usually the last resort – we get that a lot! Clients come who have tried every fad diet, every new fitness regime, and starved themselves in various ways to create a kind of yo-yo culture that plays havoc with the metabolism. None of them have brought the results they really wanted as they have failed to realise that many of the controlling decisions around their relationship to food is coming from their unregulated subconscious and they are battling against themselves – it is like their subconscious is constantly scoring own goals, and they are frustrated by themselves and their 'lack of resolve'. As a result, they are struggling with their self-image too as they feel like a failure in so many ways and so their confidence is also at rock bottom. What a difference the hypnotherapy can make to all of these issues as they find positive ways to deal with their weight issues firmly from a foundation of the subconscious supporting them from the inside out. It is truly transformational.

Mike

Mike was a fabulous teacher. He worked hard and had a way of encouraging his students to great results by inspiring them to work hard but also to love the subject of History – no mean feat these days. Mike's issue was self-confidence, as he had no idea how great he really was. I spoke to his headteacher who described him as 'one of the best – you won't find a better teacher than Mike' – but Mike could not see it himself – as with many teachers; he was his own best critic. He wanted to gain some promotion as he had worked a long time and wanted to move up into school leadership, and apparently, according to his boss he was ready. In our five sessions we were able to fill him full of positive affirmations that built up a firm foundation of confidence from the inside out. He truly started to believe in himself for the first time and was able to not only push himself into interviews, but also to secure the promotion that he desired and deserved. It was fabulous to see his progress and the respect he commanded with his colleagues and with the students. It was the power of transformational hypnotherapy for success at its best. What a great honour to work with such great people!

Mike: 'It was such a great experience – even the therapy session itself was a time of relaxation. As a teacher I never stop and certainly never get time just for me. I tried meditation in the past and it was not really for me, but hypnotherapy allowed me to take time to slow down and just catch up with myself. Then there was the confidence that I felt following the sessions. I found myself repeating my trigger word "calm" in my lessons and I noticed that I could replicate the feelings of peace and calm from my sessions and take school's ups and downs without the usual stress. I actually believed in myself enough to apply for and secure a position on SLT – the leadership team – and I had no idea I could even try out for the interview let alone get it! I was amazed how powerful hypnotherapy was; I have to admit to being a bit cynical before I tried it, but trusted Jeff enough to give it a go – and I am so glad I did! It was changed my life totally, and I would think most people could benefit greatly from giving it a go…'

'Every day, in every way, I am getting better and better'
Emile Coue

The first affirmation…and in some ways the only one that you will need to improve your life. When you take on board affirmations under hypnosis, your subconscious mind is so much more ready to accept the powerful message and start to initiate your fabulous transformation. Imagine if this was really you – every day…changes for the better each and every day… what would that mean for you? In every way – all aspects of your life; family, relationships, work, sport, arts, study… all getting better and better and more successful. Getting better and better – what would that mean for you? Finding ways to improve yourself and become the person you know deep down that you have always wanted to be…successful in the ways that you define success…finding it each day, every day in every way…is this something that you want? Hypnotherapy can allow you to achieve this faster and more efficiently than other therapies, and when combined with NLP coaching, provides a powerful package for your personal transformation.

Kathy

Kathy was dealing with stress and anxiety in her life. She was having to become a carer in her family and so had given up work to concentrate her efforts but was struggling to cope. She missed work and had not factored in how stressful doing less might be as she had worked most of her life and found this adjustment in priorities was getting her down. She said that she had always been such a positive person but that she was so frustrated with her family situation that she couldn't handle the variations of her life that that it was leaving her feeling negative and stressed out. She was anxious for no reason at small things and this was having a big effect on her general levels of confidence to keep up the job of being carer in her new situation. After a few sessions she was able to release a buried memory relating to her mum and found connections with this and her current anxiety and stress. It was a powerful and emotional release, and it was an amazing experience to be a part of such tremendous healing in this way. After the sessions she noticed that she was able to cope in new ways with her stressful situations, taking them on with ease and a realisation that she could handle anything without anxiety and stress; and claimed to be feeling confident and positive once again in her life as a whole. This was a fabulous transformation for Kathy and allowed for the possibility that anyone could benefit from this kind of therapy and find a new lease of life and positivity for their future.

Kathy: 'Thank you so much for working with me in this way; I have found a powerful release from my negativity and feel like myself once more. I had no idea just how different I could feel. I suppose on some level I had given up hope and this was a last-ditch attempt to make some kind of change in my life. When I saw your post on Facebook I had a feeling it just might be the thing and so decided to go for a consultation just to see. I am so glad I did as working with you has changed my life for the better and I am still a bit shocked as to how different I feel. I had no idea it would be so relaxing during the sessions and I feel that this is a great part of the therapy. I had been to therapy and sometimes the pressure to articulate what I was feeling was difficult and I struggled to find the release that I needed. Just sitting there and listening; then *zoning out* into my own little world while you talked was a lovely experience – so peaceful and relaxing – and I can still feel the effects now. It is such a beautiful experience that I would suggest that others have a few sessions even if they feel they have no major issues just to experience a time for themselves and find some peace and relaxation in the busyness of life. I really enjoyed it and will definitely come back for more from time to time to revitalise my life and bring my positive energy back to the forefront again. Fabulous times!'

> 'Since most problems are created by our imagination and are this imaginary, all we need are imaginary solutions'
> **Richard Bandler**

I love Richard Bandler for his tongue-in-cheek humour! He is quite the Showman! In this quote he hits on a serious note however; that most of our issues start and end in our mind. Anxiety, issues of self-confidence, our response to stress, our addictions to self-defeating practices that are destructive, our irrational fears and phobias, even our anger which is triggered by our thoughts to spark our emotions. In this sense, they are all in our imagination: the fear is not real – it is imagining what *might* happen, it triggers anxiety, stress and over-reaction causing us to become paralysed in our lives. If the subconscious creates these responses and forms the habit of poor behaviours; then the subconscious holds the keys to our release – it is in the realms of imagination as we find solutions to our problems which are based in thoughts and their entrenched patterns of negativity. NLP and hypnotherapy allow you access to your subconscious and to recreate your mind through reimagining what you want, and in the way that you would like to be in the future. Your imagination is either working for you or against you – which one will you choose? If you find an 'imaginary' solution to an imaginary problem – and you are able to live problem free – what have you got to lose but your hang-ups? Humour aside – there is a great truth here!

Melanie

Melanie was struggling with confidence and a poor self-image. She wanted to build up her confidence in order to move on from a previous partner who had left her damaged and struggling to feel good about herself and wondering whether she could ever trust another person enough to get into a relationship again. This was an extreme case of poor self-esteem and she had lost her sense of her self-concept to the extent that she was also struggling in work as she would question every decision that she made presuming it would be the wrong thing to do, and so she had been off work with stress for a few weeks by the time she came for help. During a session she found herself inside a memory of her as a baby back in her mother's arms and found such a release over feelings of abandonment and insecurity as she was healed through some inner child work and self-acceptance. After a few sessions she left looking like a new person; lighter somehow, and with a confident spring in her step. Within a few months she was not only back in work, but had gained a promotion, and was in a serious relationship that was apparently working out for her as she had found new ways of trusting herself to another person and was happy in her life. The power of the subconscious mind to know what a person needs never ceases to amaze me, and I look on this particular experience as such a learning curve as I finally understood that the subconscious really does remember everything that we do, and it knows how to release the healing when it is given permission to be in charge as the conscious relaxes itself out of the way to pave the way for transformation in a person's life. It truly is incredible!'

Melanie: 'I literally cannot believe the difference that hypnotherapy has made to my life. It is hard to explain how I feel now without getting so emotional as I recall all of the amazing changes that happened to me following the sessions. I am a new person; I am more confident that I have ever been, and I have things in my life now that I never thought was possible. It sounds ridiculous and I wouldn't believe it had it not happened to me! I had just about given up on finding my happiness – I had resigned myself to being just one of those people who has bad things happen to them and that there is nothing they can do to change. But I was so wrong! I can, and I will change as I know I can find the strength from the inside out and get release from any of my negative past. I know it can be a fantastic experience for anyone – I even enjoyed the relaxation parts, although sometimes I wasn't even sure I was being hypnotised as I was totally aware of everything that was being said to me, but I was just really, really relaxed – it's hard to describe, but it makes sense to me. I am so different now; and I really like the new me! Thankyou!'

Jill

Jill was struggling at work as she lacked confidence on the phone. She worried that others were listening in and judging her and found she would stammer when she thought about it – making it all self-fulfilling. She wanted some confidence, but also to worry less about what others were thinking about her and she wanted to feel less self-conscious in her office and wanted to get rid of the worry over what others thought about her. During our consultation it became clear that this was more than just a crisis of confidence; there were issues of identity here too going back into her past. She agreed that we would check for any possible early events that could have a bearing on her current feelings about herself and her lack of confidence. Under hypnosis she was able to discover a memory that held deep emotional ties for her and her family in the past, and when she released these memories and was able to cut them away in forgiveness and resolution, she found that her confidence grew and grew following the hypnotherapy sessions and she felt that she was a new person in some ways. She was amazed at the difference, as she had been through therapy before and had not achieved anywhere near this kind of resolution to her issues and felt that she had only 'scratched the surface' without the hypnotherapy. A bit of a cynic to start she gained a full and rich understanding of how powerful the subconscious is to create positive change or hold a person back if left in negativity. She remarked 'I can't imagine there is anyone who would not benefit from this kind of therapy – it is fantastic! I will be talking to my friends about this for a long time'. This is the power of hypnotherapy in the life of a client.

Jill: 'I can't believe the different person I have become. I just wanted to find a bit of confidence for my phone manner in my job. I did get that, but I also discovered a whole new person that I could be. I had no idea that this was even possible let alone that it could happen for me. The things that I experienced in hypnotherapy just amazed me and I was able to resolve feeling out of balance with myself and members of my family from way back, and I has made all the difference to me now. I just wanted some confidence…I didn't even believe it was the right therapy for me; yet it has changed me totally. My friends all noticed which was the best thing, and at work they can't understand how I could have had such a dramatic change in my life. They don't believe it is because of the hypnotherapy as most of them don't think that it could do any good – they have all seen the TV stuff or the stage shows that makes it all look ridiculous, and in some ways, I don't blame them –

but they have no idea how powerful it is for a source of healing, it is incredible. But they do see a different me, and at least that is something they can't deny - even though they try to make a joke out of it! I don't care, I know and that is all that matters. I really like the new me!'